Outsmart Your Fork!

Outsmart Your Fork!

A Mindful Guide To Permanent Weight Loss
(The end of yo-yo dieting!)

David Shmukler, D.C.

Mark Pustaver, D.C.

Notice

This book is intended as reference text only, not as a medical manual. The information given here is designed to help you make informed decisions about your health. It is not intended as a substitute for any treatment that may have been prescribed by your doctor. If you suspect that you have a medical problem, we urge you to seek competent medical help.

www.OutsmartYourFork.com

Dear Reader:

Just 20 years ago, not one state in the U.S. had an obesity rate over 15 percent; now there are 12 states with rates of 30 percent or more. Yet during those same years we have spent tens of billions of dollars on diets and diet books. All the expense, without tangible results, shows that diets alone don't work. We lose weight only to regain it, and then some. Since you're reading this, perhaps you can relate to the frustrating cycle of yo-yo dieting. It's time for a change! This isn't a diet book. As it says on the cover, this is a "mindful guide to permanent weight loss." The purpose of this book is to help you achieve your weight loss goals, no matter what diet plan you may be following. And much more importantly, it will serve as a guide to help you maintain that weight loss for the rest of your life.

While you can't out-exercise your fork, you can "outsmart" it, and in the pages ahead, we look forward to showing you how. Don't worry; it's easier than you might think.

David A. Shmukler, D.C.
Kennett Square, PA

Mark R. Pustaver, D.C.
Charlotte, NC

Contents

Introduction

If you've picked up this book, you probably were intrigued by its title. So was I (Dave), when it first popped into my mind. I was in the gym talking with a friend of mine who was struggling to lose weight. He had been working out regularly, but wasn't seeing results. He was getting stronger and fitter, but his weight wouldn't budge. When I asked him a few questions, his problem became pretty obvious to me. He was doing great in the gym, but the fork was still ruling his world and his weight. In fact, if anything, he had started eating more since he began working out, because the activity made him hungry, and hunger made him eat. And since he didn't know what to eat—or how much—he was, in a word, stuck. I said to him, "You know, you can't out-exercise your fork." And, unless you're an elite athlete like Michael Phelps, that's the truth. It's also the only bad news I have to tell you.

The good news is this: While you can't out-exercise your fork, you can outsmart it. The key to losing weight and keeping it off has more to do with your brain than with your body. You just need to learn how your brain works so that you can jump off the weight-loss roller coaster for good. As a chiropractor with extensive postgraduate training in neurology, I know the science behind this process, and I'll put it into terms that you don't have to be a brain surgeon to understand. As a man who has retrained his own brain to fully recover from a serious stroke, I know that brain retraining works. It's what got me from sitting in a wheelchair unable to speak to working out at the gym and being able not only to speak, but to write a book (you'll find more details about this in Chapter 1). If I could rewire my brain to bounce back from a stroke, I believe you can rewire yours to help you lose weight…or to quit smoking…or to do whatever it is you want to do.

In the pages that follow, you'll find a plan that teaches you how to "outsmart" your fork instead of letting your fork control you. No matter how long you've been overweight, you can learn to permanently control your weight, but you're going to have to do some things differently. First, you have to promise to stop dieting. People go from one diet to another, year after year. They lose weight while they're on the diet, but once they go off the diet, they gain the weight back…and then some. Diets alone don't work! Permanent lifestyle changes do. You're about to find out how to make the changes to eating behaviors and choices that will help you maintain a healthy weight for the rest of your life!

Prepare yourself to take action to "Outsmart Your Fork" today!

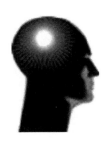

Chapter 1

How I Rewired My Brain

How I Rewired My Brain

After having a stroke at the age of 48, I taught myself to rewire my brain and fully recover.

It was April 25, 2006, and I was out for my morning run in the park. I ran for about 20 minutes, and noticed my right foot dragging a bit. I kept running, thinking nothing of it, but then I became disoriented on the trail on which I regularly run. After I finished, I returned to the YMCA for my shower. Normally, I talk to the women at the front desk, but the only thing that would come out of my mouth was a "whoosh" sound. The YMCA staff called an ambulance and though my vital signs—blood pressure, pulse, and blood sugar—all were normal, I knew something was wrong.

While I was waiting in the ER, I remembered a test I had learned to determine whether a person was having a stroke, which is when a blood vessel bursts in the brain. To test someone, you ask them to hold out both of their hands, as if they're playing an imaginary piano (kind of like an air guitar, only with keyboards). If either hand is slower or droopy or can't move, that's a sign of a stroke. Sitting there in the ER, I held my hands out in front of me and "played." My left fingers worked fine, but my right hand had slowed down. The tests the doctors gave me confirmed my suspicions: I had had a stroke.

In the days that followed, my condition worsened. When I awoke the day after the stroke, I thought that someone had cut my body in half.

I remember thinking to myself, "The right side of my body is gone!" The stroke had damaged the parts of my brain that helped it "recognize" the right half of my body. I was paralyzed on my right side and had gone from being a healthy, fit person to a totally dependent, very sick person in virtually no time at all.

While I was in the hospital, I remembered something that I had learned in my neurology training about how the brain works. It's a concept called **neuroplasticity** (NURR-o-plass-TISS-i-tee). The idea is that the pathways in your brain are actually moldable and bendable, like soft plastic. When you continue doing the same things over and over, you can change those pathways. And by changing the pathways, you change what your brain tells your body to do. Remember what your mom used to say when you'd make a face? "If you keep doing that, it'll stay that way." Turns out that she may have been (sort of) right.

So I decided to see if neuroplasticity really worked. My neurologist told me, "If you can't use your arms and legs, just visualize that you can." Several times a day, I would imagine my arms and legs moving. About two weeks after my stroke, I started to feel better. I remember telling a friend, "The fog has lifted." I made really fast progress after that. Within the next 10 days, I went from not being able to feed, bathe, or clothe myself to being able to walk and control my right hand. I was back to jogging—though in the hospital's parking lot instead of the park—less than four weeks after my stroke!

Still, I faced a long road ahead. In the months to follow I battled depression, a common occurrence for stroke victims. There were two sentences I read in the book *Feeling Good: The New Mood Therapy*, by David Burns, M.D., that started me on the road to recovery. In his book, Burns said, "Depression is not an emotional disorder, but a thought disorder. If you change your thoughts, you can change your emotional state."[1] I had used my brain to help me physically recover from the stroke; I decided to do the same to recover from my depression.

Following Burns' advice, I wrote down my thoughts, practiced meditation, changed my diet, exercised regularly, and gradually I felt better. It wasn't an overnight thing, but as time passed, I realized I was no longer depressed. I slowed down what I was doing and paid attention to my thoughts. I learned to hear what my "sabotaging voice" was saying, and I worked to change it. For example, I remember that I was starting to feel better after a few months, but then that inner voice would say, "This is only temporary; you're going to feel depressed for the rest of your life." I had to convince that negative inner voice that I was going to get better. Over the next few months I started to get control of my brain. My inner dialogue became more positive and my depression gradually lifted.

Using the same information about neuroplasticity of the brain that I used to overcome my depression, I can teach you how to retrain your thinking about food and eating behaviors. Once you gain control of that, you'll be in control of your fork. And your weight. And your body. And your life. It's a great feeling!

The first step in learning to control your brain? Understanding how this fascinating organ works.

 Mindful Thinking to Outsmart Your Fork !

- We can rewire and retrain our brain, no matter our age.

- Controlling and rewiring our brain are critical to controlling our weight.

Pause and Reflect

- Spend some time really focused on your thoughts and actions.
- Write down several key thoughts and actions that you believe are important to helping you become who you want to be.
- What do you think about practicing meditation, journaling, exercising regularly, and changing your diet in order to rewire your brain and change your life?

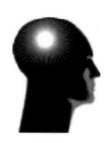

Chapter 2

The Brain-Fork Connection

The Brain-Fork Connection

Knowing how your brain and nervous system work is the first step in learning to control your thoughts…and your fork. As I mentioned earlier, to control your eating (and, as a result, your weight), you have to control your thinking. Once you understand how your brain works, that's a lot easier than it might sound. Controlling your thinking has more to do with anatomy and biology than it

> *Two simple things are key to rewiring the brain:*
> *1. Doing things differently.*
> *2. Picturing yourself doing things differently.*

does with willpower. But this isn't Biology and Anatomy 101—you just need to know enough to get by. Think of what follows as the "Quick Start" part of your brain's owner's manual. You don't need to know what all the parts are; you just need to know enough to get started on your journey to a healthier life.

Understanding your brain's "wiring"

Cerebrum. Brain stem. Cerebellum. You may have heard these "brainy" words before. But when it comes to changing a habit, it's the less famous **frontal lobe** that's the most important part of your brain. The frontal lobe is part of the cerebral cortex, which controls most of the functions that make us human. Functions like talking, thinking, remembering, creating, and analyzing all take place in your cerebral cortex. A small part of the cerebral cortex is called the **prefrontal cortex**, which controls your consciousness and self-awareness. And that's the part of your brain that ultimately can help you control your fork and change unhealthy habits into healthy ones.

Habits start when you do something regularly—like taking a walk during your lunch break, which is an example of a good habit. Each time you walk, your brain receives information about what you're doing; your eyes, ears, and nose all send messages to your brain with every stride. Your muscles and joints put in their two cents, too. Information travels through your nerves from your muscles and joints to your brain. All these things happen whether or not you consciously think about them.

Throughout your spinal cord and brain, nerve cells called **neurons** fire—"talk" to each other—as you take your walk. Although you have billions of neurons and connections, the neurons aren't directly connected to each other; there are little spaces between them called **synapses**. In these spaces, neurons release chemicals that tell the next neuron to fire or "get busy." These chemicals are called **neurotransmitters**.

The more often your neurons fire in the same way, the more connected they become to each other. It's kind of like building a friendship. The more you talk to a person, the closer you become. And the harder it is to maintain the connection if something breaks along the way, say, if your friend moves away. Neurons work the same way. Nerves that fire together, wire together. The more often nerves talk to each other, the stronger their connections become.

Although strong connections make it hard to change bad habits, strong connections can also help you create new, good habits that also can be hard to break.

The other part of your brain that plays a role in what—and how much—you eat is your **midbrain**. Your midbrain regulates your blood pressure, body temperature, and blood sugar. It's also your "emotional brain," where your pleasure centers are located. Overeating stimulates your midbrain in much the same way taking drugs stimulates the brains of drug addicts; that's how we become addicted to junk food. The food makers know this: That's why they put ingredients like sugar, fat, and salt in our food. They want to get you hooked and literally turn you into a junk-food junkie.

How to rewire your brain

Until the 1990s, it was thought that your brain was completely wired by about age four. Now we know that you can rewire your brain throughout your entire life. The technical term for the brain's ability to rewire itself is "neuroplasticity," which I mentioned in Chapter 1. There are two ways you can rewire your brain: You can do things differently over and over again until the brain rewires itself, or you can picture yourself doing things differently, which we'll get to in a minute. Let me give you a few examples of how people rewired their minds by changing what they did.

The first case involves a neuroscientist, Susan Barry, coauthor of *Fixing My Gaze: A Scientist's Journey Into Seeing in Three*

Dimensions. [2] Barry had lost her depth perception when she was an infant. Her lack of depth perception meant that when she stood on a step or a deck, she couldn't tell how far it was down to the ground. Everything in her world looked flat—like she was looking at pictures in a magazine. If she sat at a table, the tabletop looked as far away as the floor did. As you can imagine, this made her life very difficult.

At first, doctors thought Barry would never be able to regain her depth perception. Then she saw eye doctors who gave her special new exercises to rewire her brain. Barry faithfully performed these exercises over and over until one day, as she was driving home from her appointment, the steering wheel "jumped out" at her from the dashboard. She had regained her depth perception after 50 years!

Stroke patients provide us with another example of brain plasticity. Experts used to believe that, when you had a stroke, whatever you gained back in the first year or two was all the function you would ever get back. Then a study was done with stroke victims using restraint therapy. [3] Restraint therapy involves strapping down (or restraining) a patient's "good arm" and making them use their "bad arm" (the one affected by the stroke) instead. In time, most of the patients using restraint therapy regained the use of their stroke-affected arms. Also, when doctors took pictures of the patients' brains with an MRI (magnetic resonance imaging) machine, they found new connections within the brain itself. Restraint therapy had helped these patients rewire their brains.

Another real-life example involves men in their 70s. A Harvard psychologist asked one group of these men to stay in a hotel for a week. But this wasn't just any hotel: It had been changed to look as it did 20 years ago. All of the movies and TV shows the men watched were 20 years old. The music, furniture, and carpeting were from 20 years ago, too. The psychologist asked these men to live in the here-and-now and not to long for the way things used to be. A second group of men lived as they normally did. One week later, the psychologist compared the two groups. She found that those who lived in the "time-warp hotel" had less arthritis and tendonitis pain. They also had lower blood pressure. These men even looked younger! [4] Their brains had become rewired after just one week because they were constantly receiving new information. The people who kept doing the same things they always did showed no changes in blood pressure, arthritis, and tendonitis.

These examples show how you can rewire your thinking by changing things around you—things you see, feel, hear, do, and so on. The human brain is not only able to change, it enjoys changing, and it will easily rewire itself if you start doing things differently. In fact, your brain will also rewire itself if you just *picture* yourself doing things differently.

The power of positive thinking

You've heard about the "power of positive thinking"—turns out, the concept is based in scientific fact. In one study, Judd Blaslotto, Ph.D., of the University of Chicago, compared two groups of basketball players. One group spent time shooting free throws to improve their technique. A second group spent the same amount of time picturing (or visualizing) themselves shooting free throws. As expected, the group that practiced shooting free throws improved by 24 percent. But the visualization group—those who just *imagined* shooting free throws—improved by 23 percent. Just by focusing their attention, these basketball players were able to make more foul shots. [5] How was this possible? Our brains can't tell the difference between what's real and what's imagined.

Buddhist monks also understand the mind's power. University of Wisconsin researchers studied a group of these monks to see whether (and how) they could control their emotions by meditating [6]. The monks concentrated and focused on pure joy and happiness while the researchers took MRI pictures of their brains. When the researchers looked at the MRIs, they were amazed to see the part of the monks' brains that registered happiness. They had never seen people so happy! Each monk had been able to activate his brain's happiness center just by *thinking* about being happy.

Mindful Thinking to Outsmart Your Fork!

- You can change any habit or behavior anytime during your life.

- You can change habits by participating in different activities.

- You can also change habits by thinking differently.

Pause and Reflect

Make a list of your usual habits:

- What habits or patterns do you see yourself doing differently?
- What is the one thing you do now that you can change today?
- What is one thing you can change tomorrow?
- Will you spend time visualizing the changes you want to make?

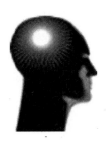

Chapter 3

The Stress-Fork Connection

The Stress-Fork Connection

Most of us live under chronic stress without ever realizing it: Joe Dispenza writes in his book, *Evolve Your Brain*, [7] that we get up in the morning, get the kids ready for school, fight traffic getting to work, answer phone calls and e-mails all day, hurry home to make meals for the family, help kids with their homework, and then go through all of it again the next day. It's enough to make you

> *Meditating, journaling, and trying new activities stimulate our brains and have a calming effect, helping to alleviate the stresses in our lives.*

feel like a hamster running on a wheel, constantly spinning without ever getting anywhere.

How much do you think about what you're doing every day? Are you just going through the motions? If you just run from one activity to the next, under stress, without thinking about what you're doing, you're in survival mode—just getting by. Chronic stress takes away our ability to think carefully about what we're doing, and as a result, we develop poor lifestyle habits, like making bad food choices and not getting enough exercise. Stress makes you crave routine. You want to do things you're familiar and comfortable with when you're under chronic stress. When you're under stress, new situations or activities can cause even more stress, so you avoid them. Doing the same negative things over and over causes negative brain plasticity (rewiring), which causes you to repeat these bad habits.

The ironic thing about getting out of this "stressed state" is that you're going to have to do the opposite of what you *want* to do to create new, healthy habits. Your emotional brain is running the show. Doing new and novel things causes you to *think* instead of *react*, which engages your frontal lobe. I remember when I was really depressed and just learning about brain rewiring. All I wanted to do was lie on the couch, stare at the TV, and eat junk food. I didn't want to see or talk to anyone. That's what I had been doing for the previous six months and I was only getting worse. I was negatively rewiring my brain, and every time I sat on the couch doing nothing but eating junk food and watching TV, I was only reinforcing negative behavior and bad habits. I had hit rock bottom and knew the only way I was going to get better was to do something different.

To help myself climb out of depression, I forced myself to go to restaurants so I would have to interact with people. I would meditate even when it was the last thing I wanted to do. I would go to the gym and work out even though my emotional brain would tell me not to go because I was too tired. Because I forced myself to get out and do new things, I allowed new and positive stimuli into my brain and created positive brain plasticity. I repeated my new activities daily. It was hard at first, but over time I felt better and gradually came out of my depression.

Each of us has an "animal brain," a pleasure center in our mind. We can stimulate these pleasure centers when we practice healthy habits, like having sex and getting enough exercise. These centers also respond to the alcohol we drink, the medications we take, and the food we eat. Unfortunately, most of the foods that stimulate our pleasure centers aren't good-for-you foods like broccoli and carrots. Instead, we tend to crave junk foods: fatty, salty, sugary comfort foods like potato chips, cheese fries, candy, and cookies.

We can become food addicts just as we can become drug addicts or alcoholics. A recent study found that food addicts exhibited the same behavior drug addicts did: They would hide big bags of candy and potato chips in drawers and closets much the same way alcoholics hide their gin and vodka.[8] When you eat that piece of chocolate cake, your brain releases dopamine, a pleasure chemical, which makes you feel better, happier. When we're under chronic stress, we look for ways to feel better, and eating junk food is just the ticket. Those good feelings make us crave more and more junk food, which becomes a vicious circle. In some ways, food addiction is tougher to conquer than other addictions, because we have to eat to live.

To fight or flee

You may have heard of the "fight-or-flight" response, which we humans developed thousands of years ago to help us stay alive in dangerous situations. In the course of everyday life, our ancestors had to decide whether they were going to run from the lion facing them or stay and shoot it. To this day, acute stress triggers the fight-or-flight mechanism in our bodies. Stress causes our brains to tell our adrenal glands to pump out adrenaline and other stress chemicals. Your pupils dilate and your heart beats faster so you can pump more blood to your muscles. You take deeper breaths. All of these processes happen very quickly. When the situation is over (and if you haven't been eaten by the lion), your brain gets feedback from your muscles, heart, and other organs to signal that the crisis is over. That's when our bodies turn off these stress chemicals.

Recent studies show that 60 to 90 percent of physician visits are stress related. [9] The chronic stresses of our daily lives continue to build because our bodies have no automatic mechanism to turn off these fight-or-flight chemicals. As I mentioned earlier, you may not even realize you're under stress. To show my patients how much stress they're under, I ask them to try to meditate for one minute. Meditation requires you to shut off your animal brain and focus on one thing; this focus takes place in your frontal lobe. Most of my stressed-out patients can't even meditate for 15 seconds! Their brains are racing with so many thoughts that they can't slow down and focus. They think it's normal to feel all keyed up. One way people handle chronic stress is to overeat. All you have to do is look around you to see people turning to food to deal with stress. I recently flew to Charlotte to meet with Mark to make the final edits for this book. In the airport I saw harried travelers eating all kinds of junk food. They were downing pastries, pizza, burgers, and candy bars. They were obviously stressed out and their food choices showed that.

Our food pleasure center and stress

The food pleasure center in your brain developed to ensure the survival of the species. For most of mankind's history, food wasn't readily available. When a person came across food, he would gorge himself because he never knew when he would find food again. Fast forward to today, when food is available 24/7 and much of what's on hand is junk food that's laced with fat, salt, and sugar. The food manufacturers know this, which is why they make all junk food with at least one of these three potentially addictive ingredients. They know you won't be able to stop eating. Remember that potato chip ad, "Betcha can't eat just one"?

Food brings us pleasure—just what the "animal" part of our brain looks for. And because we don't always wait for hunger, we often eat when we're happy, sad, bored, or depressed. Most of us eat for emotional reasons and aren't even aware of what these reasons are. It's only when we become self-aware that we will eat for the right reason (when we're hungry). If you primarily eat to give your body the nutrition it needs, you can create a healthy habit. If, on the other hand, you eat every time you feel bored, lonely, depressed, or stressed, you can create an unhealthy habit. A friend who is following our program said, "I was unaware of how unaware I was." He had developed the habit of eating a whole bag of pretzels at night without thinking. Eating these huge amounts of food was just part of his routine. Now that he's more self-aware, he measures out a 200-calorie serving of pretzels. By regularly eating more mindfully, he has rewired his brain.

Self-awareness: The key to permanent weight loss

The longer you live under chronic stress, the more you'll use your animal brain to seek pleasure and the less you'll use your frontal lobe to focus on what you're really thinking and feeling. Stress causes us to react without thinking and makes us do things absentmindedly. That's why it's so important to develop self-awareness to activate your frontal lobe and start thinking again. You can develop new habits anytime if you want to.

One way to combat stress is to become more self-aware. Now that I'm self-aware, I know why I'm overeating; it's mainly when I'm tired or bored. Before I became more aware of why I ate, I would eat a decadent lunch and dinner every Friday. I wasn't thinking about what I was doing; it was Friday and that's just how I ate. Now I go for a swim at

Developing greater self-awareness is an important step in combating stress, rewiring our brains, creating new healthy habits, and gaining control over our fork.

lunchtime; the exercise releases the same pleasure chemicals food does. Do I eat junk food occasionally? Yes, I do. But now I realize I'm eating it and know when to stop. *I'm* in control, not the chemicals in my brain. Now that I'm more self-aware, I'm able to recognize my boredom and steer myself toward healthier activities that keep me from eating (like writing a book).

Mindless unhealthy eating → Mindful healthy eating →Mindless healthy eating

Our goal is to move from mindless unhealthy eating (like going into the kitchen four or five times a night and grabbing junk food out of the refrigerator or pantry, even though you're not hungry) to mindful healthy eating (consciously eating the same breakfast every day and eating primarily when you're hungry) to mindless healthy eating (healthy eating habits that have now become automatic and so routine in your life that you no longer have to think about them).

It takes 60 to 90 days of focus and self-awareness to create new eating habits. [10] This is the mindful phase, when you're developing self-awareness. It's when you go on a diet, eat what you're told, and follow a plan. But diets only take you so far. If you can stay motivated until you form a healthy habit, then you've got it. You no longer have to stay motivated to brush your teeth, for example, but when you were first developing that habit, your mom probably reminded you to brush each morning and night. Once you think about what you're doing, like eating more healthfully, consuming more good-for-you foods will become a positive habit, just like brushing your teeth. You don't think "I have to brush my teeth today," you just do it. That's the same thing you can do with your eating habits.

One of my physician friends lost 35 pounds and has kept it off for 15 years. His secret? He weighs himself every day. If he gains a couple of pounds, he knows he has to be careful about what he eats. He's in control, not his fork. He also eats the same healthy lunch and breakfast during the work week; he doesn't have to think about what to eat, he already knows what he's going to have. His eating has become a mindless healthy habit.

I practiced a mindless unhealthy eating habit for years. I would work out every morning, and then head to the local convenience store to buy a newspaper and a bag of peanut M&M's. That would be my breakfast most days. I wasn't thinking about what I was eating; I just ate it. When my coauthor, Mark, was doing nutrition research, I became more self-aware. I said to myself, "Why am I eating M&M's for breakfast?" With my newfound self-awareness, I changed what I ate and have now eaten the same healthy breakfast for two years. I eat a whole grain cereal, banana, almonds, and blueberries. That's a much healthier breakfast and I don't even have to think about it. I just do it. I have created a mindless healthy habit. Do you have an unhealthy eating habit?

How you can become self-aware

Once you become more self-aware, it's relatively easy to change your habits and rewire your brain. No matter how long you've been overweight, you can get control of your fork and your weight—but you need to *want* to do it. Even if you've had a weight problem for many years, have "bad genes," and engage in bad stress-related habits, you can overcome all of that by becoming more self-aware.

Self-awareness lowers your stress chemicals and is a sign of a healthy frontal lobe, the part of your brain that allows you to make decisions.

There is a close relationship between your frontal lobe and your animal brain; that connection happens in the part of your brain that releases stress chemicals. When you think clearly and make decisions, your frontal lobe signals to your animal brain, telling it, "We've got this, we're in control." The result: Your animal brain turns down the level of stress chemicals. On the other hand, when your animal brain is in control, it sends signals to your frontal lobe that make it harder for you to think clearly.

When I was depressed, I had a hard time making even the smallest decisions. My animal brain had effectively shut off my frontal lobe. Once you become more self-aware, you'll notice its effects in many parts of your life. You won't just make healthy food choices; you'll also make healthy life choices.

For example, I was in a minor car accident recently and had a chance to use my newfound self-awareness. Instead of getting worked up like I used to, I remained calm. I made sure no one in the other car was injured. I had a notepad in my car and wrote down all of the insurance information. I was in control. If this accident had occurred a couple of years ago, I would have yelled at the other driver and probably would have forgotten to write down the information. It would have ruined my entire day. Instead, the accident was a relatively minor inconvenience. The better way I handled this situation demonstrates how healthy my frontal lobe is. When you have an experience like this, pretend you're a fly on the wall, impartially observing the situation. That will help you use your frontal lobe to *think* about the situation instead of reacting as you may have done hundreds of times in the past. Being self-aware helps you rewire your brain and create new healthy habits.

The only way you can change a behavior is to become aware of what you do, such as when you eat and what you feel when you eat. Here are some strategies to get you started.

Keep a food journal. To become more aware of your eating habits, I recommend you use a food journal to write down what you eat. Be honest; keep track of every morsel of food that passes your lips and everything you drink that isn't water. You may also want to write down what you're feeling when you eat so you can become aware of the moods and feelings that lead you to overeat. Also make note of who you are with and where you are so you become more aware of situations that cause you to make unhealthy choices. When you reflect back on the past week, can you think of a time when you overate? If so, can you associate it with a "trigger" that caused you to lose control over your fork? Part of the process of becoming more mindful is to become aware of the triggers that affect your eating, whether they are a person, a place, or an emotion.

Weigh yourself every day. It's easier to lose a pound or two than it is 20 or 30 or more. When you weigh yourself every day, you'll be able to catch any weight gains early so you can do something about them. A daily weigh-in will reinforce the self-awareness you've developed.

Meditate. Meditation has a soothing and calming effect on the pleasure center (your animal brain) and is probably the best way to become more self-aware. Meditation involves focusing on just one thing for as few as 12 to 15 minutes a day. Meditation can help you make permanent brain changes by engaging your frontal lobe, which gets bigger and functions better with daily meditation.

One study proves my point nicely. Researchers recently divided college students into two groups. One group meditated for 12 to 15 minutes a day for eight weeks, while the other group went about their normal routines. After eight weeks, scientists looked at the students with functional MRIs. (Like regular MRIs, functional MRIs show three-dimensional pictures of the physiology of your brain. Functional MRIs also show which parts of your brain are more active.) In the non-meditating group there were no brain changes, but the meditation group showed evidence that their frontal lobes had become rewired—they had actually grown new brain cells, making their frontal lobes thicker! This study shows that we can make profound changes to our brains in as few as eight weeks. [11]

Most of us are taught that we're products of our genes and our environments. If both of your parents are overweight and you have had a stressful life, it does not mean you are destined to be fat. This study and many others have found that you can change your brain by what you think. A healthier frontal lobe helps you think and make decisions more clearly. You'll be more self-aware and make better food choices. You can overcome a lifetime of bad behaviors just by thinking differently.

Change your daily routine. Practice activities that force you to pay attention to what you're doing and put you in the moment, like brushing your teeth and combing your hair with your non-dominant hand. If you don't concentrate on brushing your teeth with your "other" hand, you'll get toothpaste all over your face and body. Driving a different route from home to work also requires you to focus your attention. Because it's a new activity, you can't put yourself on autopilot: You have to concentrate, just like when you first learned how to drive. You can also "turn on" your frontal lobe by engaging in any kind of new activity, like learning how to play the piano or speak a foreign language. These new activities force your brain to make healthy new connections. Remember, your brain rewires itself for a lifetime as long as you continue to try new things: Think back to those gentlemen in their 70s who lived in the "retro hotel" for a week (see Chapter 2). What have you done lately that you've never tried before? Go for it. New thoughts and new activities will lead to new emotional experiences. [12]

I see this all the time when my patients go on vacation. Going on vacation, particularly to a place you've never been, forces you to try new things in a non-stressful environment. A friend of mine went to Hawaii recently and every day was filled with new activities, from zip lining to hiking to sight-seeing. He also shut off his phone so he couldn't receive any e-mails from work. His brain got a lot of new input and he felt great! When he returned I had never seen him so relaxed. So please try something new. You'll feel better than you've felt in years and will be in control of your emotional brain instead of letting it control you.

Don't forget to move. Physical activity is good for your brain—especially cardiovascular exercise. Whatever exercise you choose, it has to be something you like to do and can enjoy doing regularly over the long haul. You shouldn't exercise because your spouse or children want you to; you should exercise because *you* want to. When you exercise to please someone else, it becomes just another form of chronic stress and you won't benefit from positive brain changes. I enjoy running and have some of my greatest insights when I'm out jogging. Running "reboots" my brain and helps me think much more clearly.

Get plenty of sleep. Getting enough sleep is important to your brain as a whole and to your frontal lobe in particular. Not getting enough sleep and feeling tired all the time can signal to your brain that you're hungry. Simply put, your brain needs to be satisfied. If it isn't getting enough quality sleep, it seeks satisfaction elsewhere. Most people will turn to junk food to satisfy their cravings. I know when I'm tired, I crave junk food. Now, instead of eating, I take a 20-minute nap to refresh me.

Chronic stress can wreak havoc on your sleep. Before my stroke, I would fall asleep within a minute of my head hitting the pillow. For a long time after my stroke, though, I had great difficulty sleeping; the stress chemicals from my animal brain wouldn't shut off. Do you remember the "fight or flight" response we talked about earlier in this chapter? If you were running from a lion, you would feel very alert and under acute stress. My chronic stress made me feel like I was running from lions all night instead of sleeping! Now I am back to sleeping as I used to. Every night before I sleep, I meditate. Meditation makes me feel calm so I can get seven or eight hours of uninterrupted sleep.

Keep a mood diary. I also recommend you keep a mood diary to increase your self-awareness. As you write down how you feel before, during, and after you eat, you'll begin to see trends and will be better able to pinpoint those situations and feelings that make you eat when you aren't hungry.

An example of a mood diary can be found at the end of this chapter.

Build a support network. It's very important to have people who can support you on your weight loss journey. They can help relieve the stress by showing you that you are not going through these changes alone. In moments of weakness it's important to have someone to talk to, someone who can help you stay on track. I was a member of a running group for many years. There were days I didn't feel like running, but I knew other people would be there and were depending on me. Other runners would tell me that if I hadn't been in the group they wouldn't have run on certain days. Being part of a group makes you accountable to other people. Some days you're going to lift them up when they're under stress, and other days they'll be the ones to help you. Of greatest importance is having the support of your spouse or partner and any other individuals living with you. Life, like our refrigerator, is full of temptations, and you need to have the support of those closest to you in order to have the greatest success in your journey to mindless healthy eating.

Mindful Thinking to Outsmart Your Fork!

- Chronic stress causes us to develop many poor habits, including unhealthy eating. We're most likely unaware of these bad habits because we've been doing them for such a long time.

- We have no built-in mechanisms to turn off chronic stress. The key to turning off stress is self-awareness.

- There are many ways to develop self-awareness, including meditation and exercise.

- Learning new skills helps your brain grow. Try something new like learning a foreign language, playing a musical instrument, or simply changing your daily routine.

- Keep a mood diary to pinpoint feelings (or any sabotaging voice) that may cause you to eat when you aren't hungry.

- Get seven to eight hours of sleep a night.

- Build a support network to help you reduce stress and reach your goals.

Pause and Reflect

- Think about the mindful thoughts and lifestyle tips from this chapter. Are you willing to make a commitment to incorporating them into your daily routine, to help you achieve your weight loss goals and to enable you to live a longer, healthier, more active life?

MOOD DIARY

Date: ___/___/___

Time: _____ AM/PM (please circle one)

Craving: __ Starch __ Sweet __ Salty __ Crunchy __ Other (specify)

_____

Alternatives to eating: __ Meditate __ Walk __ Lift weights __ Hobby

__ Other exercise (specify) _____

__ Other activity (specify) _____

Mood before you eat: __ Happy __ Sad __ Stressed __ Angry __ Anxious __ Bored

__ Other (specify) _____

Mood while you're eating: __ Happy __ Sad __ Stressed __ Angry __ Anxious

__ Bored __ Other (specify) _____

Mood after you've eaten: __ Happy __ Sad __ Stressed __ Angry __ Anxious __ Bored

__ Other (specify) _____

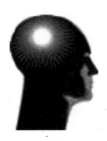

Chapter 4

The Food-Fork Connection

The Food-Fork Connection

The diet industry is a $50-billion-per-year industry. According to the Centers for Disease Control and Prevention (CDC), obesity caused by unhealthy diet and lack of exercise kills 400,000 people a year. If spending money on gimmicky diets were the answer to obesity, we would have solved the problem by now.

Every year new diets come out, people lose weight while they're on them, and then gain back all the weight—and then some. Ninety-five percent of all people who go on diets gain the weight back. Why? They don't make the mental shift toward permanent weight loss. To maintain weight loss, you have to continue good eating habits for the rest of your life. But the first thing most people do once they've reached their goal weight is to revert back to their old habits. Any diet works when you're counting calories and eating a strictly regimented meal plan. But if you don't become self-aware while you're developing these new habits, you'll be yo-yo dieting forever. When you don't address the core issues, you don't become self-aware. You need to develop a lifetime plan for permanent weight loss.

> *To achieve our weight loss goals and, more importantly, to permanently maintain a healthy weight, we need to develop "mindless" healthy eating habits, be self-aware, and keep chronic stress in check.*

The 5 percent of people who do maintain their weight loss have become self-aware and are able to keep their chronic stress and weight in check. They have developed healthy "mindless" habits that will last the rest of their lives. These people also use tools such as keeping track of what they eat (food journaling) and weighing themselves every day to stay on track. I'm going to give you the tools you'll need, so you won't have to go on any more diets. You'll still be able to eat chocolate, ice cream, and other favorite foods, but *you* will be in control. Before I give you the tools, though, you need to know the basics of nutrition.

Nutrition 101

Calories are a measure of how much energy your body uses. You must burn 3,500 more calories than you consume per week to lose one pound. You'll have to burn 500 more calories each day or eat 500 fewer calories each day or a combination of the two (500 calories multiplied by 7 days a week equals 3,500 calories) to lose a pound of weight. Your body's metabolism also plays an important role. Each one of us has a different metabolic rate—the number of calories you have to eat each day to maintain your current weight. If you're a sedentary person, you need approximately 12 to 13 times your body weight in calories each day to maintain your weight. If you're an active person, on the other hand, you'll need approximately 15 times your body weight in calories. For example, a sedentary man weighing 165 pounds would need to eat approximately 2,000 calories a day, while an active man would need to eat about 2,500 calories a day just to maintain his current weight. [13]

For a healthy diet, you should eat nutritious food that fuels your body. The best fare includes whole foods such as fruit and vegetables, beans, and whole grains. These foods are nutrient-dense, which means they're rich in vitamins, minerals, fiber, and other nutrients. Junk food is calorie-dense, which means it contains few vitamins and nutrients, but lots of calories. Since junk food stimulates your brain's pleasure centers, it's easy to overeat it.

Calories in, calories out

You could eat any food and lose weight as long as you eat fewer calories than you burn up. For example, one study found that a man who ate mostly Twinkies, along with other junk food, lost 27 pounds in 10 weeks. Before you run out and buy cases of Twinkies, though, keep in mind that he was eating 1,800 calories a day of mainly junk food, but his body needed about 2,600 calories a day: He was burning more calories than he consumed. The calories he ate just happened to come from junk food. [14]

This eat-what-you-want concept is what's behind many gimmick diets like the cookie diet, the smoothie diet, the grapefruit diet, and others. In fact, I could eat only peanut M&M's and still lose weight. Junk food contains very few nutrients, vitamins, fiber, or antioxidants. If you eat whole foods such as fruits, vegetables, and whole grains, you're eating foods that make you healthier and that are associated with a lower risk of heart disease, diabetes, and cancer. Plant-based foods also contain no cholesterol. You also could eat only organic, natural, low-fat food and still gain weight. If you burn more calories than you consume—from any food—you'll lose weight. On the other hand, if you eat *more* calories than you burn, you will gain weight. In order to keep the food-in/calories-out equation operating in your favor, you need to have tools in place so you're aware of what—and how much—you eat.

People go on gimmick diets year after year because they haven't made the mental shift to permanent weight loss. They think, "I lost 40 pounds on the Smoothie Diet last year, so I'll just go on it again and lose the weight." They repeat the same thing over and over and expect a different result. The diet companies know this and every year come out with the "new and improved" Smoothie Diet. Unless you develop self-awareness and adopt new healthy habits, you may be going on the "Super Peanut M&M's Diet" next year!

When people go on diets and eat the same amount of calories, they can lose different amounts of weight depending on how active they are. Trouble is, most people can't lose weight by exercise alone without changing what they eat, too. You may think that if you exercise, you don't need to be aware of what (and how much) you eat. It's great if you exercise regularly, but that's only half the equation. I see people in my office who exercise regularly but are still overweight. They aren't aware of what they're eating.

Unless you're mindful (aware) of what you're putting into your mouth, your fork will always win. You can exercise for a half hour every day and burn up 300 calories per session, but if you're still eating an extra 300 calories that day, your weight won't budge. A recent government study found that an average woman has to exercise one hour per day just to maintain her body weight! That means she's eating approximately 500 calories per day more than she needs to. If you have to exercise an hour a day just to maintain your weight, you're eating too many calories. An hour of exercise will likely burn 500 calories depending on the activity and intensity. If you're trying to lose weight, you can either exercise more or become more self-aware about what and how much you're eating. (The study also mentioned that if these women changed their diets they wouldn't have to exercise as much.) [15]

The bottom line: Weight loss is really very simple. You have to burn more calories than you consume. Here are some tips that will lead you to greater self-awareness and a whole new way of living.

Keep track of your calorie consumption. Write down what you eat and drink or use a smart phone application to track calories (some apps also allow you to track your mood). Some of these smart phone applications take less than two minutes a day. If you plan ahead of time what you're going to eat each day, you put your mind in control, not your emotions. No matter what kind of day you've had, just follow what you've written down for your meals ahead of time and you'll stay in control. When you keep practicing these healthy eating behaviors over and over, they become habits—mindless, healthy habits.

Tune in to your mood. Take a minute before you eat and ask yourself:

- Am I making a healthy food choice?

- Am I really hungry and fueling my body?

- Am I eating for an emotional reason?

- Am I tired, bored, anxious, happy, depressed, lonely, or something else?

The more you ask yourself these questions, the sooner you'll begin to realize why you're overeating. If you identify that an emotion is the trigger, and not actually hunger, you'll find a healthier way to treat the emotion—by meditating, journaling, exercising, etc.

Create a healthy environment. If you can, remove all the junk food from your house. If that's not possible, make portion-controlled bags of your favorite junk foods so you know how much you're consuming. I know I have a weakness for peanut M&M's, so I don't keep any in my house. (Remember: The foods that stimulate the pleasure centers of our brains are salty, sugary, and fatty.) I keep only whole foods in my house, including fruits, vegetables, beans, nuts, whole grain cereals, and lean meats.) If you were an alcoholic trying to kick the habit, you wouldn't keep beer in your house. If you were trying to quit smoking, you wouldn't walk around with a pack of cigarettes in your pocket. You want to make creating new habits as easy as possible, and remove any temptations.

the solution

One key to creating a healthy environment is to make a shopping list of healthy foods when you're at home. Once you're at the store, stick to your list. In general, the healthiest foods are in the outer aisles, so stick to the perimeter as much as possible. Don't give in to the temptations of the center aisles, which can be a junk food extravaganza!

Give it time. Remember that it takes two to three months of practicing a new activity almost every day to create a new habit. Now that I'm self-aware, if I want some chocolate I go out and get the smallest bag of candy (250 calories) and eat it. I can still enjoy chocolate but I don't gorge myself. A friend of mine, who has a "movie night" with his wife, weighs out his candy before he goes to the movies. He's in control. Recently, though, I overheard a man in a restaurant who was clearly not aware of the lifestyle choices he was making. The man was eating a big bowl of pasta with meatballs and sausage. His friend asked him, "Don't you have high cholesterol?" The man replied, "Yes, I do, but my doctor put me on a statin [a cholesterol-lowering drug] so I can eat whatever I want." It's hard for most people to change long-standing habits.

Go beyond exercise. Another friend had recently moved to California and was fortunate enough to be able to take a year off from work. He was exercising four or five hours per day but the weight was coming off slowly. I asked him, "Why isn't the weight coming off faster, if you're exercising like crazy?" He said, "Dave, you can't out-exercise your fork." His cupboard and refrigerator were full of all kinds of unhealthy junk food. He was unable to control himself. He was probably burning more than 3,500 calories a day and eating about the same amount. He hadn't developed self-awareness and hadn't created an environment for weight loss. His words stuck with me and became the basis for this book.

Eat the same breakfast every day. This creates positive brain plasticity. Remember that we are trying to create healthy mindless habits. You're repeating a good new habit over and over. If you made some bad food choices the day before, the next morning get right back on track. As I mentioned earlier, I eat the same thing for breakfast every day, so I don't have to think about what I'll eat.

Don't waste calories on sodas and juices. I drink mostly water. If you eliminated two sodas a day from your diet and didn't do anything else, you would lose about 20 to 30 pounds in one year! Sodas are one of the worst things you can consume, because they're almost pure sugar and just empty calories. Juices are obviously much more nutritious but contain a lot of calories, too. It's better to eat a piece of fruit—you'll get fiber, nutrients, vitamins, and fewer calories. If you do drink diet sodas, just remember that even though they contain no calories, they may cause you to eat more. Diet drinks trick your brain into thinking you're eating something sweet and can lead to cravings for junk food. You have to be self-aware when you drink diet sodas.

Focus on good health. We're trying to give you weight loss tools for the rest of your life so you don't need to go on any more diets. You'll also be healthier when you lose weight and may not have to take as many drugs for conditions related to your poor lifestyle habits. This is not about how you look, it's about being healthy. Remember, we want to take you from mindless unhealthy habits to mindful healthy habits to mindless healthy habits.

Make small but lasting changes. Eliminate sodas, eat the same healthy breakfast every day, eat more fruits and vegetables, plan out your daily meals ahead of time, and weigh yourself every day to put yourself in control. You'll need some monitor or gauge to show that you're staying on track. Seeing the dentist every six months is a gauge you're taking care of your teeth properly. Likewise, you need a daily gauge for eating properly. If that means you have to weigh yourself every day, or keep a daily food journal on your smart phone for the rest of your life, that's what you have to do. These changes don't require a big time commitment; they take only a few minutes a day and after a while you will do them automatically! They become part of your routine.

The difference between our permanent weight loss lifetime plan and any reduced-calorie or fad diet you try is that our plan contains no gimmicks. There are no magic potions to buy. You're not going to have to go on a new diet next year. You just have to keep practicing the new habits you've learned and keep a check on your stress levels. If you keep trying new diets without becoming more self-aware of what conditions make you eat and which foods tempt you, you're going to be on and off diets for the rest of your life. That's what the

Simple!

another whole matter!

multibillion-dollar diet industry wants you to do so they can get you to try their "diet du jour." If you're more self-aware and use the tools we offer here, you won't have to play the diet game.

The one thing I can tell you for sure is that stressful situations will come up in your life. I hope that your new self-awareness will help you recognize these situations so you won't have to turn to food for comfort. Of course, everyone makes bad food choices sometimes. But when I make bad food choices, they end at breakfast the next day, because I automatically weigh myself each morning and eat the same healthy breakfast. If I gained a pound or two from my out-of-control eating, I write down what I'm going to eat that day. I know if I eat more fruit, salads, and vegetables, I'm usually back to my desired weight in a couple of days. Compare that to most people who can't gain control over their weight. An anesthesiologist friend told me that most of his patients in their 50s are 30 to 40 pounds overweight and take cholesterol, blood pressure, and diabetes medications. These diseases are largely lifestyle diseases—the result of the American lifestyle, which combines chronic stress, overeating, and being sedentary.

If you had a stressful day that led to mindless unhealthy eating, remember that tomorrow is the dawn of a new day, and you can get back on track with your usual healthy breakfast.

If you ever feel tired of weighing yourself or writing down what you eat, it's usually a sign that you're under stress. ("My life is too busy already, and these are just two more things I need to do!") Feelings like this mean your emotional brain is in control again and you're back to turning to food for comfort. When you get to these stressful points in your life, it's important to have developed self-awareness, which will help you recognize what your stressors are. If it's your family or work, you can address the issues instead of avoiding them and turning to food for comfort. You may have to talk yourself through it or reach out to a family member or friend, someone who can support you on your healthy lifestyle journey. Everybody goes through these moments of weakness. Being self-aware will help you get right back on track.

 Mindful Thinking to Outsmart Your Fork!

- To increase self-awareness, you have to keep track of what, when, and how much you eat.

- Eat the same healthy foods for breakfast every day.

- Eat whole foods such as lean meats, fish, beans, fruits, whole grains, vegetables, nuts, and seeds.

- Don't drink your calories; eliminate sugary sodas from your diet.

- To lose weight, you have to burn more calories than you take in, no matter what kind of calories you eat (fat, carbs, or protein).

- Limit the amount of foods you eat that are processed with white sugar, white flour, saturated fat, and artificial sweeteners.

- Plan your daily meals ahead of time to stay in control, and stick to your shopping list.

- If you consume dairy products such as milk, cheese, and yogurt, choose low-fat or nonfat varieties.

- Weigh yourself every day to catch any weight gain before it gets out of control.

- Form a support network of family and friends to encourage you to stay on track.

Pause and Reflect

As you've read this chapter, can you relate to any of the unhealthy, "mindless" eating habits? Will you commit to replacing those old habits with new "mindful" healthy habits?

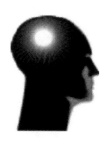

Chapter 5

The Fit-Fork Connection

The Fit-Fork Connection

You've probably heard that exercise holds many health benefits—it's good for your bones, heart, muscles, and brain. Cardiovascular exercise, in particular, has been shown to help create brain plasticity (rewiring). As good as it is for you, you may not

> *You can't out-exercise your fork, but exercise will help you develop a happier brain and a healthier body.*

like to exercise. That's why it's so important to choose a workout routine you enjoy—something you'll be able to fit into your lifestyle. If you exercise because you feel you *have* to (rather than *want* to), it will cause stress and won't lead to the positive brain changes you're aiming for. Exercise has to be your choice to reap the positive brain benefits.

Healthy brain changes from exercise include growing new brain cells (neurogenesis), improving memory, and even helping to overcome depression. Regular exercise stimulates your brain and helps combat stress. If you're a "stress eater" this is critically important because you have a healthy way to stimulate your brain instead of turning to junk food.

Exercise needs to be part of your lifetime plan, not just part of a 10-week diet. You can incorporate exercise into your daily routine by taking simple steps (no pun intended) like taking the stairs instead of using the elevator. Keep your walking shoes in your car; if you have a half-hour lunch break, take 15 minutes and go for a walk.

Just one simple strategy can help you start burning more calories: Buy a pedometer. These simple gadgets are inexpensive and easy to use. Shoot for a goal of 10,000 steps a day (about five miles), which burns on average 300 to 400 calories. The idea is to get moving, because your body is meant to move. If you limit your calorie consumption but you're still not losing weight, you may not be getting enough activity. At the end of the day, write down how many steps you've taken, which will make you more aware of your activity level.

Many good exercise programs are available, from Latin dance, step aerobics, tennis, and spinning classes, to more solitary activities like swimming, walking, running, and weight lifting. You could look into joining a local gym if you'd like to participate in group exercise. I like to lift weights, run, and swim, and on most days I'm doing one of those activities. I prefer working out in the morning before I go to work; that way, no matter what comes up during the day I've already exercised. I don't even have to think about it: As soon as I get out of bed I automatically head to the gym or to the running trail. I've created a mindless healthy habit, and I've maintained this habit for years.

It's important to choose a time when you can exercise regularly and to pick an activity you enjoy. Choosing an exercise routine you enjoy is especially important when you're just starting to exercise, because you're trying to create a healthy habit. It's much easier to form a habit if you're doing something you like.

Once you've picked the time of day to exercise, decide for what amount of time you want to be active. I recommend 20 to 30 minutes a day to start. If you have time, you can build up to an hour a day. As you become more fit, you should be able to increase the intensity of your workout and not have to increase the amount of time you spend exercising. It's important to increase your intensity as exercise becomes easier for you, because you'll burn more calories and see greater changes in your body as you exercise harder. Of course, before beginning any new exercise program, you should first consult your doctor.

Recently, scientists asked people who stood on their feet all day at a retail job to switch to a sedentary desk job. In six months the average study participant gained 18 pounds just from the decreased activity! [16] It's a balance of two factors: how much you eat and how much you move. The people in the study were eating the same amount of calories but burned about 300 fewer calories a day when they started desk jobs.

As you become more self-aware, you can use exercise to combat your emotional eating. I used to eat when I was bored, now I exercise instead. Exercise stimulates your brain and releases feel-good chemicals. If you continue to exercise when you're bored—or for whatever emotional reason—you'll create a mindless healthy habit.

Beginner exercise program

When it comes to exercise, you'll find an almost endless variety of activities from which to choose. Join a local health club to find an exercise program that's right for you. In the following pages, we offer you a simple 20-minute exercise program for beginners. Our exercise program will incorporate cardiovascular (heart-strengthening) exercise and weight training. You'll exercise six days a week— walking three days and lifting weights three days. It's important to remember that you need to increase the intensity of your workout as you become more fit. Choose a time of day you can exercise regularly so it becomes a mindless habit.

The only equipment you'll need for our exercises are a good pair of walking or running shoes and a set of light dumbbells (a weight you can lift for 10 to 12 repetitions) or power bands to provide resistance.

If you keep following the program for a full 10 weeks, you'll eventually move into the mindless healthy habit phase.

Walking program

Week 1

To start, just walk on level ground or set your treadmill to a low level for 5 minutes. If you have a heart rate monitor on your treadmill, use it. It's good to exercise at 75 percent of your maximum heart rate. If you don't have a heart monitor, that's fine; you can estimate 75 percent of your maximum heart rate using the "talk test." If you can carry on a conversation easily, you're walking too slowly. If you're so out of breath you can't talk at all, you're walking too fast. When you can respond with some difficulty, you're walking at the perfect intensity. [17] Warm up slowly for 5 minutes, train at 75 percent of your maximum heart rate for 3 minutes, then go down to 50 percent for 2 minutes. If you don't have a heart monitor, just estimate 50 percent of your perceived maximal effort. Repeat. Walk another 3 minutes at the 75 percent level and 2 minutes at the lower level. Do this for 20 to 30 minutes. Keep track of how far you go. Walk using these directions 3 days your first week. Walk every other day. As you get more fit you'll walk farther and faster.

To summarize week 1:

- Warm up slowly for 5 minutes.

- Train at 75 percent of your maximum heart rate for 3 minutes.

- Go down to 50 percent for 2 minutes. (If you don't have a heart monitor, just estimate 50 percent of your perceived maximal effort.)

- Repeat the first 3 steps: Walk another 3 minutes at the 75 percent level, then for 2 minutes at the 50 percent level.

- Continue this for 20 to 30 minutes. Keep track of how far you go.

Week 2

Walk 4 minutes at 75 percent of your maximum heart rate and 1.5 minutes at the 50 percent level. Repeat. Walk for 20 to 30 minutes 3 days this week.

Week 3

Walk 5 minutes at your 75 percent level and 1 minute at the 50 percent level. Repeat. Walk for 20 to 30 minutes 3 days this week.

Week 4

You may be in such good shape that after the warm up, you'll be able to walk the entire 20 to 30 minutes at your 75 percent level. Walk 3 days this week. If you can't walk at that speed for that length of time, don't worry; just walk for as long as you can at the higher level.

Write down how far and how often you walk to keep track of the progress you make. If you walk three times a week, you will have formed a mindless habit. Exercise will be part of your new healthy lifestyle!

Weight lifting program

For the following 20-minute weight lifting program, you'll need light dumbbells or resistance bands, an exercise mat, and a sturdy chair. Count to 3 in each direction of the exercises. By doing this, you'll work your muscles both ways and see more benefits from the exercises. As the exercises get easier, increase the weight you use. As you become more fit, try to do 2 or 3 sets of each exercise. If you're just using your body weight for an exercise, you obviously can't increase the weight, so just do more repetitions.

Warm up. The purpose of warming up is to get your blood flowing. Walk in place or on the treadmill for 3 minutes. Stop walking and do 20 windmills with your arms in each direction. Then do 10 torso rotations in each direction. (Twist at the waist while standing up straight.)

Half squats. Stand on the floor in front of a chair with your legs hip-width apart. Keep your back straight, lower yourself for a count of 2, and just touch the chair with your bottom but don't fully sit down. Return to a standing position. Do 1 set of 15 repetitions. Do not let your knees go over your toes. Bend at your hips, not at your knees.

Push-ups. Lying face-down on the floor, do 1 set of as many pushups as you can. If you can't do regular pushups, get on your knees and do pushups from that position, which makes it easier. If you can't do either form of pushup, lie on your back, holding a dumbbell in each hand. Push the dumbbells away from your body and return. Just be sure to choose a weight you can lift 20 times.

Biceps. Hold both arms down at your sides with your palms facing forward and a dumbbell in each hand. Flex your elbow and bring the weight up as far as you can. This works the biceps muscle. Do a set of 15 flexes (curls) and remember to count to 3 in each direction, up and down. Do 1 set of this exercise.

Triceps. Grip a light weight (a weight you can lift 15 times) with both hands. Extend your arms over your head. Bend at the elbows back toward your head as far as you can (keeping your shoulders still) and then return to the extended position. Repeat 15 times. Do 1 set.

Shoulders. In each hand, grab a light dumbbell. Lift the weight to shoulder height with your palms facing away from you. Extend your arms over your head as far as you can and then return them to shoulder height. Look straight ahead while you are performing this exercise. Count to 3 in each direction. Do 1 set of 15 repetitions.

Abdominals. Lie on your back on a mat. Hold your hands behind your neck. Bend your knees with your feet flat on the floor. Tighten your abdominal (stomach) muscles by bringing your shoulder blades off the floor. Don't pull on your neck. Hold for a count of 2. Repeat 15 times.

Mindful Thinking to Outsmart Your Fork !

- Exercise has many health benefits, including positive brain effects. These include growing new brain cells, improved memory, and combating depression.

- Pick an exercise you enjoy and a time of day you can exercise most days of the week. Make regular exercise a habit.

- Start walking at least three days a week, eventually building up to taking a daily walk.

- Buy a pedometer and write down your activity level to boost your self-awareness.

- If possible, create a standing work station.

Pause and Reflect

Stop for a moment and think about the level of physical activity you've achieved this week:

- Could you have found time to exercise more?
- What exercise(s) do you most enjoy?
- In the upcoming week, what time and days will you plan on doing that exercise?

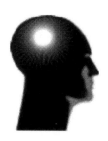

Chapter 6

Your 10-Week Healthy Lifestyle Plan

Your 10-Week Healthy Lifestyle Plan

Most people who go on diets fail. No matter what diet you try, there's a 95 percent failure rate. People tend to go on diets until they reach their goal, and then revert back to their old eating and lifestyle habits. Another reason people fail? Stress. When

> *The "Outsmart Your Fork!" 10-Week Plan will help you to rewire your brain and develop mindless healthy eating habits that will become permanent and enable you to live a healthier, more active life.*

you're under stress you have a tendency to revert to your old habits. If you've had a habit for 30 years, it's almost "hard-wired" into your brain. But as you learn new eating behaviors, you create new habits and change your brain's wiring. At first, these new, healthy brain pathways aren't as strong. Your old (bad) eating pathways are similar to a four-lane highway, while your new pathway is like a trail you're trying to cut through the jungle. When you're under stress, which pathway is going to be easier to travel? That's why you're going to have to develop safety checks for the rest of your life that will keep you from reverting back to your old eating habits. You'll need to gauge your daily stress, just as your car's gas gauge tells you when it's time to get gas.

During these 10 weeks, we'll give you a step-by-step plan to gain control of your fork and your life. In the process, we're going to make it as easy as possible for you to rewire your brain. Remember, the goal of this 10-week program is to develop mindless healthy habits. We'll try to motivate you through these 10 weeks, but motivation only goes so far. The key is to repeat the same new activities and behaviors over and over until they become habits. Think of it this way: You don't have to be motivated to brush your teeth every day, you just do it. Brushing your teeth doesn't take willpower, because it has become a healthy habit. The healthy breakfast I enjoy every morning has nothing to do with motivation; it's a habit. In fact, one of the things we recommend in our healthy lifestyle plan is that you eat the same healthy breakfast every day.

I'll guide you through what, and how much, you should eat to make it easy for you. I'll ask you to keep track of what you eat (food journaling) and weigh yourself every day starting from day one to help you build self-awareness. I'll ask you to practice these new habits until you do them without thinking. Daily meditation also will be part of your healthy routine. Our program, which includes meditation, food journaling, and exercise, will take you about 30 to 45 minutes a day. Is it worth it? We think so—unless you want to stay on the diet merry-go-round.

You will be eating the same breakfast every day. Examples of healthy breakfasts are oatmeal, cold cereals, fruit, raw nuts, and so on. Pick something you like to eat that's healthy. You're going to gradually switch what you eat to whole foods (fruits, vegetables, lean meats, beans, and whole grains). You can make these foods tasty without adding a lot of fat or salt. If you're bored eating the same breakfast every day, I would argue that you're probably eating the same food every day *now*, but it is junk food, not healthy food. The difference between our program and other diets is that we're not just telling you what to eat and how much, we're also giving you tools to develop self-awareness so mindless healthy habits become part of your life. We want to make these new habits as routine as brushing your teeth, so you don't even have to think about them.

Discover your purpose

When I had my stroke and was lying in the hospital bed, I had plenty of time to contemplate my purpose. I couldn't walk, couldn't use my right arm, and had great difficulty speaking. The nurses' aides bathed, fed, and clothed me—all things I used to take for granted. In this totally dependent state, I remember saying to myself, "I want to recover so fully that I'll have to tell people I had a stroke. I want my telling them to be the only way they'll know." Now people are shocked when I tell them the story.

When Mark's daughter was born, he told me that "with her first breath, she gave me a profound purpose in life." We all need to find our "profound" purpose for developing mindful eating habits and maintaining a healthy weight.

That was my purpose. What's yours? Why are *you* taking this weight loss journey? Your purpose has to be meaningful. Your purpose may be that you want to set a good example for your family or to become healthier. Maybe you want to stop taking (or take less) medication for diabetes, high blood pressure, or cholesterol. Eating fast food only occasionally would be a great first step in easing your need for diabetes, blood pressure, and cholesterol-lowering medications. A British cardiologist once suggested that when people eat at a fast-food chain they should be given cholesterol-lowering medication with their orders. [18] I can see it now: "I'll have a double burger with cheese, large fries, a large cola, and 40 milligrams of Lipitor. He was dead serious because we Westerners love fast food.

You must want to lead a healthier lifestyle for yourself, not because someone else is forcing you, otherwise it just becomes another stress in life. And if your purpose is too shortsighted, like wanting to lose 30 pounds for a wedding, you won't make the mental shift to a lifelong habit. How many times have you seen people lose weight for a wedding, class reunion, or other "important" event? They look great at the event but when you see them a few months later you hardly recognize them, because they have gained all the weight back, and then some. Losing weight for a wedding could be a smaller goal within a more meaningful purpose. Was there a time you lost weight for an "important" event, only to gain it back afterwards? If so, don't feel bad; most of us have. I would encourage you to find a deeper, more meaningful purpose. Examples of such purposes would be: "I want to be able to play with my children and grandchildren." "I want to take fewer medications and not feel tired all the time." "I want to blow out the candles on my 100th birthday cake." Choose a profound and long-lasting purpose.

Now that's a big purpose!

Rhonda has been overweight all her adult life. Over the years, she gained and lost the same 50-100 pounds countless times. She would be motivated to lose weight for a wedding or some other event, only to regain the weight shortly afterwards. Once again, Rhonda was on a diet, but she told me _this_ time she would keep the weight off for good. Why would it be different this time? She went on to tell me she was recently diagnosed as having a severe heart condition, one that was due in large part to her obesity. She said her doctor told her, "If you don't lose weight, you are going to die!" Now that indeed is a big purpose!

Outsmart Your Fork ! 10-Week Healthy Lifestyle Plan

Mindless unhealthy eating → Mindful healthy eating → Mindless healthy eating

Week 1

1. **Write your purpose on a slip of paper.** Tape it to the refrigerator and add it to your smart phone.

2. **Weigh yourself every morning** (ideally, for greatest accuracy, using a digital scale that measures in tenths of a pound). We know most people don't want to get on the scale, but it's an important step to becoming more self-aware. You have to know what's working for you and what isn't. Don't let your emotions get the best of you, and don't be afraid—it's just a number.

3. **Write down (journal) what and how many calories you eat every day** in a notebook, or input the number of calories into your smart phone.

4. **Eat the same healthy breakfast every day.**

5. **Build a support network.** It's much easier to reach a goal when a friend or family member encourages you. It's even better if your friend makes lifestyle changes with you. There are days where you're going to need help; make

sure you have someone to count on. It makes the journey much easier when you have people to share your experiences with, and to encourage you in times of weakness.

6. **Take "before" pictures of yourself from the front and side** in shorts and T-shirts. Keep the pictures in your phone or on your refrigerator. You should also post a picture of yourself when you were thinner or at your ideal weight to stay focused on your goal.

We'll give you more tips over the next 9 weeks but the first five above are the most important, so you must follow them every day. Remember, you're on the journey from mindless unhealthy habits to mindful healthy habits to mindless healthy habits. These 10 weeks are the mindful phase of your weight loss journey, so you'll need willpower and discipline. You'll have to tell yourself, "This is what I'm going to eat today." You won't be able to let your emotions tell you what you'll eat.

If you keep following the program for the full 10 weeks, you'll eventually move into the mindless healthy habit phase and you will arrive at the point where you get more enjoyment out of feeling good than eating bad.

Week 2

1. **Meditate at least once a day for 10 to 15 minutes.** Meditation is the best way to develop self-awareness. The

best times to meditate are either first thing in the morning or before you go to bed. The meditation technique we recommend for beginners is called "focused attention" and is outlined in *Relaxation Revolution*, by Herbert Benson, M.D. [19] Close your eyes and focus on your breathing. Feel the air go into your nose and mouth, breathe slowly, and count your breaths. Stay in the moment and note how your body feels. If other thoughts pop into your head (and they will) just be aware of them and go back to counting your breaths. The longer you can focus on your breath, the calmer you'll feel. Don't worry if the first few times you meditate you can't do it for longer than a minute or so. Meditation takes practice, just like learning any new skill.

Focusing your attention daily is one way to manage chronic stress. Keep practicing and meditation will get easier. As it gets easier, you'll be able to focus on other relaxing things when you meditate, like your favorite vacation spot where you can picture yourself on the beach. Try to hear the waves crashing or watch the seagulls. What beach smells do you notice? Your brain can't tell if you're in Hawaii or if you're just imagining you're there. Just think: You'll be able to take a vacation every day, even if it's for just 10 minutes and in your mind. Imagine how much better you'll feel when you go on your family vacation if you meditate every day. Your stress level will be much lower and it won't take you three or four days to unwind. You'll enjoy your vacation from day one.

2.   Continue the healthy habits from Week 1.

Week 3

1.   **Throw out all the junk food in your house**, if possible. If that's not possible, keep portion-controlled bags of your favorite snack foods handy, which will make it easier to create new healthy habits. Remember, we have to create a healthy environment.

2.   **Slow down - you move too fast**. At least when it comes to eating, many of us do. Relax and chew your food longer and more slowly. Be aware of the taste and texture of the foods that you're eating. Give yourself time to savor and enjoy your meal. When you eat more slowly, it gives your stomach more time to tell your brain that you're full. By slowing down and focusing on what you're eating, you will actually eat less and feel more satisfied.

3.   Continue the habits from Weeks 1 and 2; they should be getting easier for you. Continue meditating. You should start to feel more relaxed. If you're following an eating plan, you should have lost some weight and you are starting to gain control of your brain.

Week 4

1.   **Keep a mood diary** (see Chapter 3). When you crave a food, write it down. What emotion is associated with that craving? Are you bored, anxious, or tired? Participate in another activity besides eating to stimulate your brain. Go for a walk, exercise, read a book, play a computer game, or call a friend. If the craving is too strong to fight off, find a healthy alternative snack like nuts or fruit. When you have a craving that won't go away, it usually means you're under stress, and you'll be tempted to eat unhealthy food. But you don't have to resort to junk food! As you develop greater self-awareness, you'll realize that stress can signal it's time to take a walk.

2.   **Eat your fruit, don't drink it.** Replace juices, sodas, and milk with water. Fruit juices are high in calories. Whole fruits also contain fiber, which keeps you feeling fuller, longer.

3.   Meditate and focus on your purpose every day.

4.   Weigh yourself daily.

5.   Continue your healthy habits from the previous weeks.

Week 5

1.   **Buy a pedometer.** See how active you are by writing down how many steps you take each day. Try to build up to 10,000 steps a day.

2. **Find and start an exercise program you'll enjoy.** Do it the same time each day so it becomes a habit. Join the local fitness center or gym; see if they have any programs you'd like to try. There are many exercise DVDs that feature lots of different types of exercise. We have a beginner exercise program in this book if you don't know how to get started (see Chapter 5).

3. Continue to write down what you eat, weigh yourself every day, and continue to meditate. Remember that you're in control.

Week 6

1. **Eliminate animal products from at least one meal a day.** If you eat the same healthy breakfast every day that I do, you've already accomplished this. Many studies show the benefits of eating more vegetables, whole grains, and fruit. [20] Beans are a good source of protein and are low in fat, and you can substitute them for meat in many recipes.

2. Continue to journal, meditate, exercise, and weigh yourself every day. You may notice the benefits of self-awareness in other aspects of your life, too. You may feel calmer, make better decisions at work, and have more patience with your kids. You'll probably also sleep better and feel less tense and anxious. You should also feel healthier, be

losing weight, and feel like you're gaining control over your fork.

Week 7

1.   **Focus on 80 percent.** Every time you eat a meal, say to yourself, "I'm going to eat until I'm 80 percent full." (This comes from the Japanese saying "hara hachi bu.") If you say this at every meal, it's another way to reinforce your newfound self-awareness.

2.   **Stretch out your meditation.** Meditation has probably started to become easier for you and you can likely do it for longer periods of time. You look forward to meditating because it relaxes you. You don't have to drink coffee every morning to get you going or have a drink at the end of each day to calm you down. You don't feel under as much stress. By this time, your emotional brain has calmed down and you're using your frontal lobe to act, rather than using your emotional brain to react.

3.   Continue with your other healthy habits from the previous weeks.

Week 8

1.   **Expand your horizons.** Stimulate your mind with a new activity. Try a new exercise. Give yoga or Pilates a try, take Ballroom Dancing lessons, or start playing tennis. If you're mountain biking or running, find a new trail to

travel. If you've never played an instrument before, it's never too late to learn. Challenge your mind with crossword puzzles or begin playing chess. Check out your Community College for classes that might be of interest to you. Learn a new language. Plan a trip to a destination you've never been to before. If that destination is a foreign country, a great combination would be to begin to study and learn the language of that country before you take your trip. It's time to discover and try new things.

2. Continue all of the behaviors you've been practicing for the past seven weeks. These should continue to become easier to implement.

Week 9

1. **Go natural.** Eat mainly whole, unprocessed foods, such as fruits, vegetables, beans, lean meats, nuts, and whole grains. If you don't understand the ingredients on the label, don't eat the food. Remember, though, that even if you eat whole foods, you still need to pay attention to portion sizes and calories. High-fiber foods fill you up and keep you feeling fuller, longer.

2. Remember, you can change your lifestyle anytime you want to. We're giving you the tools to do just that. Keep up with your weekly habits.

Week 10

1.   **Congratulate yourself!** By now, you should be more self-
     aware and should have developed the mindless healthy
     habits you can carry with you for the rest of your life. No
     more diets. You weigh yourself, write in your food journal
     every day, and keep track of what works for you. On the
     days when you eat fewer refined sugars and starches (like
     those in cookies, candies, cakes, and bread), you'll lose
     weight. Your pedometer will keep you aware of your daily
     activity. You should be meditating daily without even
     thinking about it. When you're at parties, you know what
     to eat and how much. If you get on the scale the next
     morning and you're up a pound, you don't panic. You get
     back on track by eating the same healthy breakfast you've
     eaten for the past nine weeks and vow to eat fewer starchy,
     sugary, and fatty foods that day. The next day you'll be
     back to where you want to be. You will have outsmarted
     your fork!

Outsmart Your Fork ! Mindful Eating Plan

The self-awareness you've learned will help you through this 10-
week program. You'll eat the same healthy breakfast every day. Does
that mean for the rest of your life you have to eat the same foods for
breakfast? Yes, on most days you will, and you won't even need to
think about it. Occasionally, I eat a different breakfast if I'm out of

town for a day or two. Then I go back to my same breakfast and continue weighing myself every day. I'm still in control. When you don't want to eat your healthy breakfast, it usually means you're under stress. I hope that with the self-awareness you've developed, you'll know what your stressors are and find another way to deal with them besides eating. If you can do that, you will have benefited from our program and made a healthy lifestyle change.

Our 10-week plan will work with any diet. Any diet program works when you're disciplined and eating what you're supposed to eat. We're trying to give you the behavioral tools so you won't yo-yo diet for the rest of your life. It always comes down to calories burned versus calories consumed.

For those of you who are not following a specific diet plan, what follows is a sample daily meal plan. We've set the daily caloric intake at approximately 1,500 calories. Depending on your starting weight and activity level, your specific caloric needs may be more or less than this. You will likely lose between one and three pounds a week for the first few weeks. You'll notice that the breakfast we suggest is the same breakfast I eat. If you don't like cereal, you can pick any breakfast you like that's nutritious and contains about 400 calories. If you eat snacks, be sure to write them down in your food journal. Try to keep your snacks to no more than 100 to 200 calories. As you plan your meals, keep in mind that meats and cheeses are very high in calories and fat.

Every weekend, plan your meals for the following week. Go grocery shopping and get all the items you'll need. Each day, look at your food journal or your smart phone to see what you'll be eating that day. After you eat your meal, write down what you actually ate. With smart phone apps, planning ahead should take you no more than a couple of minutes a day. Taking the time to plan puts you in control. If you find that one particular lunch and dinner works better for you, repeat it. Remember, we're in the weight reduction and mindful stage (willpower and determination). Once we go into the mindless healthy habit phase, you'll be able to eat more depending on your activity level.

Sample daily eating plan

Breakfast: One cup of shredded wheat, half a banana, half-cup of blueberries, 10 almonds, and half-cup of milk. Calories: 340

Lunch: A 100-calorie sandwich thin with 1 slice of tomato, 3 ounces of sliced deli meat turkey breast, mustard, lettuce, and tomato. One apple. Calories: 400

Snack: 20 raw almonds. Calories: 140

Dinner: One grilled chicken breast, salad with 2 tablespoons fat-free Italian dressing, 1 cup broccoli, half-cup brown rice. Calories: 450

Salads should include as many vegetables as you like (spinach, peppers, carrots, and so on). The more brightly colored vegetables, the better. Vegetables are nutritious, high in fiber, and low in calories. Even better, they fill you up. I recommend using a low-fat or nonfat dressing. Make sure you measure the dressing because they contain lots of calories.

Dessert: 1 medium peach and nonfat yogurt. Calories: 160

Daily calorie total: 1,490

A note to vegetarians and vegans: You can substitute beans and soy products, quinoa, and brown rice for animal products.

Remember to eat the same healthy breakfast each day to create a mindless healthy habit. If you have too many choices, it's easy to overeat. These next 10 weeks are going to be important to break your unhealthy eating habits. These weeks will put you in control, but will take willpower and self-discipline. But if you follow this program consistently, you'll develop the mindless healthy habits that you'll take with you for the rest of your life. No more dieting!

 ## Mindful Thinking to Outsmart Your Fork !

- The keys to permanent weight loss are the action steps we outline above. The most important tips include weighing yourself every day, eating the same healthy breakfast, food journaling, and meditation.

- It takes most people 10 weeks to create a new habit. When you perform these action steps daily, you create mindless healthy habits.

Pause and Reflect

- Will you commit to this 10-week plan?
- Are you willing to do what it takes to make permanent lifestyle changes?
- Will you begin today to create mindless healthy habits?

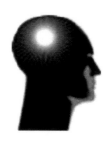

Chapter 7

Outsmart Your Fork Forever!

Outsmart Your Fork—Forever!

The main thing I want you to take away from reading this book is that

> *Stay on track to maintain a healthy weight for the rest of your life!*

you can change any habit at any time in your life if you want to. It was quackery just a few years ago to think you could rewire your brain and, as a result, change any behavior. Now, with new imaging tools such as MRIs, we can show that your brain does change if you do new things repeatedly. In this book, I've shown you how to control your weight for the rest of your life by rewiring your brain. And I've given you simple tools to help you become more self-aware.

It's common to see people lose a lot of weight and gain it all back. Often, the reason they gain it back is because they don't have a way to monitor their chronic stress, let alone do anything about it. Chronic stress is insidious—it just creeps up on you. You have to make sure you don't fall prey to its detrimental effects. If we didn't face chronic stress, it would be easy to change our behaviors and keep the weight off.

When you reach your goal weight and have developed mindless healthy lifestyle habits, keeping the weight off seems easy, because you're doing what works best for you. You need at least two or three action steps to help you keep your weight in check for the rest of your life.

As I wrote about in earlier chapters, I have three steps I continue to use daily:

- I eat the same healthy breakfast;

- I weigh myself every day; and

- I meditate.

I can tell you without question that meditation has made the biggest difference in my life. I'm calmer, more relaxed, and think more clearly. I can look at the scale and recognize that if I'm up a couple of pounds it usually means I have some stressor in my life that I need to address.

If you don't have a gauge to keep track, you won't know whether you're in control of your stress and your weight. If you get tired of weighing yourself every day, it usually means you're stressed out and your emotional brain is taking over. If you are not weighing every day, it is likely because you are afraid of what the number on the scale will be. Summon the courage and take the small step up onto the scale and get back in control of your health. Here's a tip: Try to be an impartial observer of yourself when you look at the scale. Look at your scale the way you look at your gas gauge. You don't get emotional when you're running low on gas (unless you run out); you just go to the nearest gas station.

If you've gained a few pounds over a weekend, just look at the scale on Monday and plan out your meals for the next couple of days and do the action steps that you have learned worked for you. Observe your situation without all the drama. Because we're usually stressed out, most of us often only look at our situations without seeing other options. We become self-consumed. With self-awareness, you'll be able to look at your life situation differently and stay in control of your fork and your life.

When we were children many of us were afraid of the "monster hiding in the closet," a dreadful being that put fear in our hearts and minds. It seems for some of us, the scale is the adult version of that monster, something that can't actually hurt us, yet we fear it. Just as we overcame the fear of that monster by confronting it when our parents opened the closet door and showed us there was nothing to be afraid of, so it is with weighing ourselves. We

> *For many of us, the scale is the adult version of the "monster in the closet" that we were afraid of when we were children.*

have to step on the scale and confront our fears. When you weigh yourself for the first time, if the scale reveals you weigh more than you expected, allow yourself one minute to deal with any guilt, frustration, or anger, then forgive yourself and begin your journey to reaching a healthy weight. An important point to keep in mind is this: We weigh what we weigh, whether or not we know the number. The scale gives us knowledge, and in our quest to becoming more self-aware, as the saying goes, "knowledge is power."

Big Bob

Mark recently shared with me a conversation he had with one of his patients who was starting a diet. At 6'7" and almost 400 pounds, you'd think Big Bob wouldn't be afraid of anything, yet he was intimidated by a 2" high scale. Mark told Bob that it would be beneficial for him to weigh himself every day, but Bob said he couldn't do that because it was too "emotionally difficult." Mark recommended to Bob that as difficult as it can be, he needed to look at weighing himself more analytically. He told him to think of weighing like a science project; each time you weigh, whether you go up, down, or stay the same, you think about the day before, and analyze how your body reacted to what you had to eat and drink, and how it responded to your level of physical activity. Think about the stresses and situations of the prior day, and how they affected your eating. Mark went on to explain that weighing daily is all about increasing our awareness. So as challenging as it can be to overcome the anxiety and fear of the scale, it is an important step in learning the "science" of our bodies.

We need to reframe our thinking when it comes to the scale and weighing ourselves every day. Not only is the scale a very beneficial tool in our quest to reach and maintain a healthy weight, it can also be a great motivator. As we lose weight we'll get the positive feedback and reinforcement every time we weigh ourselves. This is extremely motivating and will give us encouragement to stay on track. On the days we don't lose weight, or perhaps even gain weight, we can then evaluate what occurred and how we ate the day before, and make the necessary changes.

I understand that your life will sometimes be stressful. That's why it's so important to find ways to combat that stress. In this book, we've given you the tools to stay in control for the rest of your life. Is it worth half an hour a day to use these self-awareness tools? It is for me.

Follow this 10-week program and the lifetime plan, and you will have solved your weight problem once and for all. You will be off the diet merry-go-round for good. That's a great feeling!

You must want to change, and now you can because we have given you the tools. I watched a TV documentary about weight loss recently. An obese man repeatedly went to a prominent university's inpatient weight loss center for weeks at a time, where he spent thousands of dollars. After his last visit he said, "I finally realized I'm going to have to do it." By that he meant he needed to implement the new habits he had learned and practice them daily. He needed to develop self-awareness.

There are plenty of diets and drastic invasive measures to help combat obesity. Diet gimmicks, medications, and gastric bypass surgeries are all available. Far too often we look outside ourselves for a quick fix, but **the answer lies within**. All we need to do is be mindful, change our brain, and outsmart our fork.

Memorize these two sentences

Mindful Thinking to Outsmart Your Fork !

Congratulations! You now have the daily self-awareness tools to lose weight and manage chronic stress:

> ➢ Meditate.

> ➢ Keep a food journal.

> ➢ Weigh yourself every day.

> ➢ Eat the same healthy breakfast every day.

- Chronic stress is insidious and may cause you to revert to your old habits. You have to use the daily tools to keep stress and your weight in check.

- It's vital to have a big purpose and people to support you.

- Read this book every three months to motivate you and to remind you of all the healthy habits you have learned.

Pause and Reflect

You now have the information and tools to begin living a more mindful and healthier life. We invite and encourage you to begin your journey today.

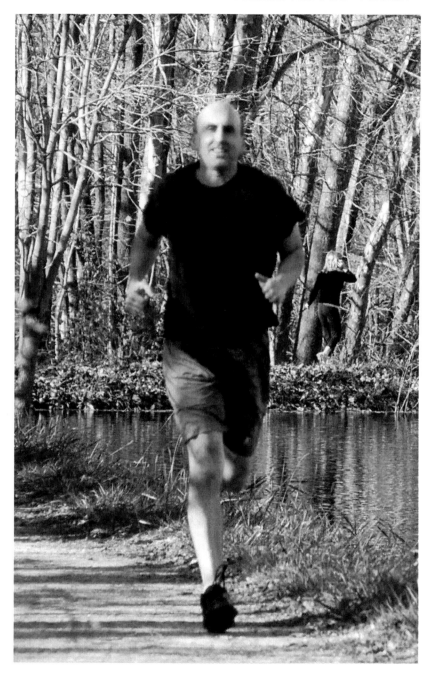

Photo by Jim Waters

Dave – November 2011

Acknowledgements

I want to first express my gratitude to Dave for inviting me to join him in writing this book. Since he first called me and asked if I wanted to work with him on this project, it has been a most interesting, enjoyable, and stimulating experience. In the book, we discuss the benefits of doing new and novel things. Writing this book has certainly been that for us and being able to write it with a friend makes it even more special.

Dave and I would like to thank Frederick Carrick, D.C., Ph.D., for it was "Ted" who first enlightened us about the concept of neuroplasticity.

Several individuals have given us much appreciated guidance in writing and editing this book. Laura Quaglio's input has been extremely valuable. Not only did she help edit the book, she gave us guidance in focusing our writing on a brain-based approach to dieting. We are grateful to Linda Rao and Karen Kenney for their editing skills. We also thank Mary Lawing for her talent and creativity in designing the cover of this book.

Many friends have given us encouragement and advice along the way. We want to thank Mike Guglielmo for his support and incredible enthusiasm in this project. We also want to thank our friend Tom Kelly, M.D., for it was Tom's comment to Dave that "you can't out-exercise your fork" that planted the seed to write a book. Dave would also like to express his personal gratitude to his dear friend Barb Lent. Barb was there to give Dave her support and encouragement in those most difficult days after his stroke and in the challenging months during his recovery. He is eternally grateful.

Growing up, both Dave and I were fortunate to have loving, supportive parents who gave us guidance and the confidence that we could achieve anything we wanted in life. We'd like to express our tremendous appreciation and love to our parents: Dr. Nathan and Joann Shmukler, and Dr. Frank and Gayle Pustaver. Dave would also like to thank his siblings, Lori, Steven, and Gail Shmukler, and I'd like to thank mine, Gregg and Dana Pustaver and Vicki Sharpee. We realize the importance of a support network, so it is truly a gift to have the love of siblings as you go through life. We'd like to make a special thank-you to my sister Vicki, who found the time in her very busy life to offer us her perspective, expertise, and suggestions that we believe helped to make this a better book.

I want to thank my wife, Myra. Being the wife of a doctor can be difficult at times, as our schedules can be rather demanding. When one adds writing a book into that schedule, life gets even more hectic. Myra's love, understanding, and support through this process were truly appreciated. I am blessed to have her in my life. More than anything else, I'm grateful to Myra for the gift of our daughter, Alexandra. As it says earlier in this book, with her first breath, Alexandra gave me a profound purpose in life.

Lastly, Dave and I would like to thank you for choosing to buy this book. There are countless other diet-related books you could have selected, so we are grateful you have chosen to "Outsmart Your Fork!"

Mark R. Pustaver, D.C.
Charlotte, NC

Appendix

1. Burns, David D., M.D., *Feeling Good: The New Mood Therapy*, William Morrow and Company, Inc., 1980.

2. Barry, Susan R., *Fixing My Gaze: A Scientist's Journey Into Seeing in Three Dimensions*, Basic Books, 2009.

3. Taub, E. Morris, D.M., "Constraint-Induced Movement Therapy to Enhance Recovery after Stroke," *Current Atherosclerosis Reports* 3(4):279-286 doi:10.1007/s11883-001-0020-0, 2001.

4. Langer, Ellen J., Ph.D., (2009). *Counterclockwise: Mindful Health and the Power of Possibility*, Ballantine Books, IBSN: 978-0-345-50204-9.

5. http://www.breakthroughbasketball.com/mental/visualization.html "Mental Rehearsal & Visualization: The Secret to Improving Your Game without Touching a Basketball!"

6. University of Wisconsin-Madison, "Compassion Meditation Changes the Brain," *Science Daily*, March 27, 2008.

7.   Dispenza, J., *Evolve Your Brain*, pp. 254, Health Communications, Inc., 2007.

8.   Society for the Study of Ingestive Behavior, "Evidence for 'Food Addiction' in Humans," *Science Daily*, July 12, 2011.

9.   http://www.pbs.org./tcc/headlines headlines_health_mind body.html. " The Mind- BodyConnection"

10.   Lally, P., van Jaarsveld, C.H.M., Potts, H.W.W., and Waddle, J., "How are habits formed: Modeling habit formation in the real world," *European Journal of Social Psychology*, 40:998-1009 doi:10.1002/ejsp.674, 2010.

11.   http://www.ncbi.nlm.nih.gov/pubmed/21071182 – "Mind fulness Meditation Leads to Increases in Gray Brain Matter in Just 8 Weeks"

12.   Dispenza, J., *Evolve Your Brain*, pp. 194, Health Communications, Inc., 2007.

13.   http://en.wikipedia.org/wiki/Basal_metabolic_rate

14.   http://www.cnn.com/2010/HEALTH/11/08twinkie.diet.pro fessor/index html.

15.   Lee, IM, et al. "Physical activity and weight gain prevention," *JAMA* 2010; 303(12): 1173-1179.

16.   Boyce, Robert W., et al. "Physical activity, weight gain and occupational health among call centre employees,"

OccupMed (Lond) 58 (4): doi:10.1093/occmed/kqm135, 2008.

17. http://www.unm.edu/~lkravitz/Article%20folder/talktest.html

18. http://www.dailymail.co.uk/health/article-1302544 would-like-statins-fast-food-outlets-hand-cholesterol-drugs.html.

19. Benson, Herbert, M.D., and Proctor, William, J.D., *Relaxation Revolution: The Science and Genetics of Mind Body Healing*, Scribner, New York, 2010.

20. Campbell, T. Colin, and Campbell, Thomas M. II, *The China Study: The Most Comprehensive Study of Nutrition Ever Conducted and the Startling Implications for Diet, Weight Loss, And Long-Term Health*, BenBella Books, 2006.

About the Authors

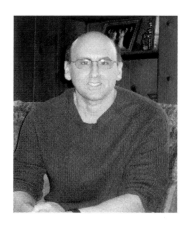

David Shmukler, D.C., graduated from the National College of Chiropractic with the Doctor of Chiropractic Degree, receiving a B.S. in Biology from Juniata College prior to his doctorate degree. Dr. Shmukler has lectured to the public and physicians about chiropractic, including a multi-disciplinary group in Mission Viejo, California on "Whiplash Injuries". He has extensive postgraduate training in neurology and enjoys sharing the concept of "neuroplasticity" with others. He lives and maintains a private chiropractic practice in Kennett Square, PA.

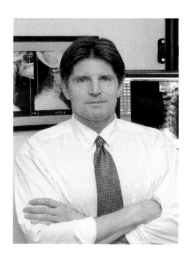

Dr. Mark Pustaver is a Board Certified Chiropractic Neurologist and Certified Chiropractic Sports Physician. He serves as a Team Chiropractor for Hendrick Motorsports and the Chiropractic Consultant for the Charlotte Bobcats. He is in private practice in Matthews, NC. He lives in Charlotte, NC with his wife, Myra, and daughter, Alexandra.

We can rewire and retrain
our brain. Brain plasticity.
Use your frontal lobe. Think
instead of reacting.